All by myself

PANTS, VEST, GETTING DRESSED!

First published in paperback in 2015 by Wayland

Copyright © Wayland 2015

ISBN: 978 0 7502 9620 5
Library eBook ISBN: 978 0 7502 7268 1
10 9 8 7 6 5 4 3 2 1

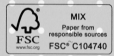

MIX
Paper from
responsible sources
FSC® C104740
FSC
www.fsc.org

Printed in China

Wayland
An imprint of Hachette Children's Group
Part of Hodder & Stoughton
Carmelite House
50 Victoria Embankment
London EC4Y 0DZ

An Hachette UK company
www.hachette.co.uk
www.hachettechildrens.co.uk

All photography by Adam Lawrence except
p1tr: iStock; p4tr & l, 5, 8, 9, 12, 13, 15tr &bl, logo and all backgrounds: Shutterstock

All by myself

PANTS, VEST, GETTING DRESSED!

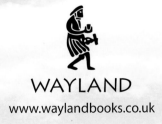

WAYLAND
www.waylandbooks.co.uk

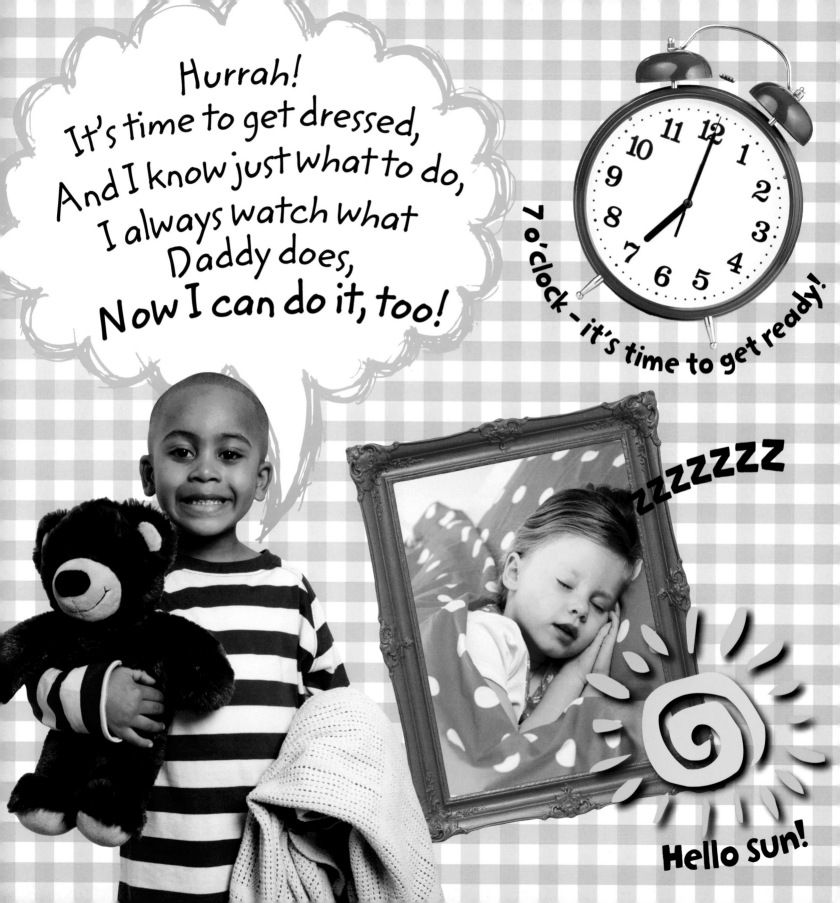

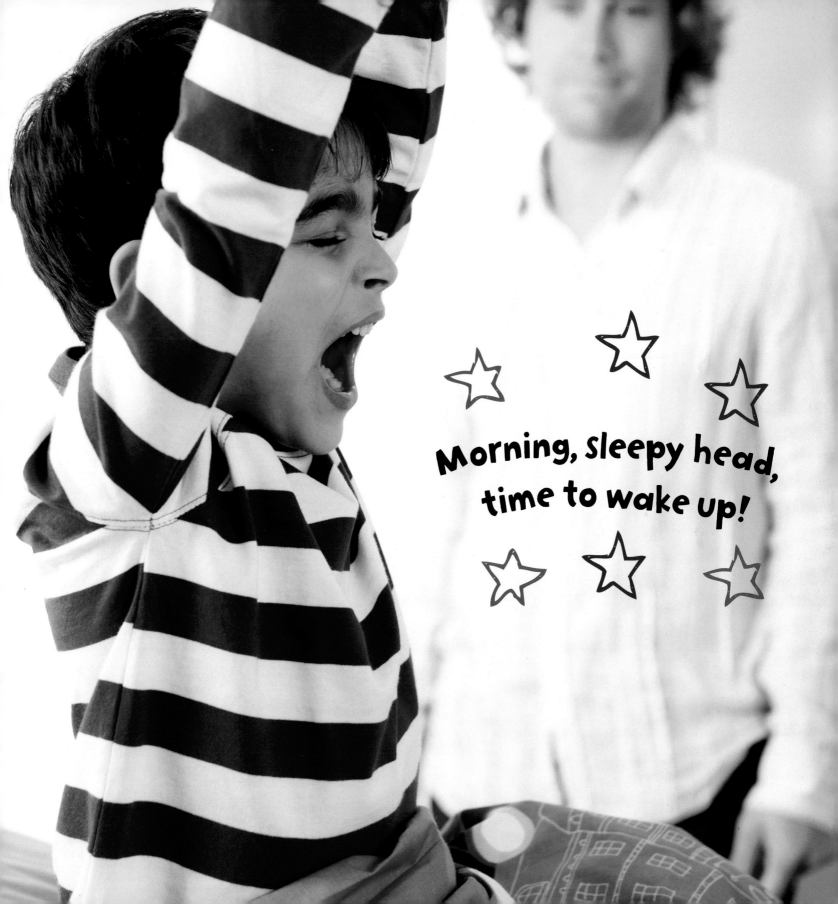

Morning, sleepy head,
time to wake up!

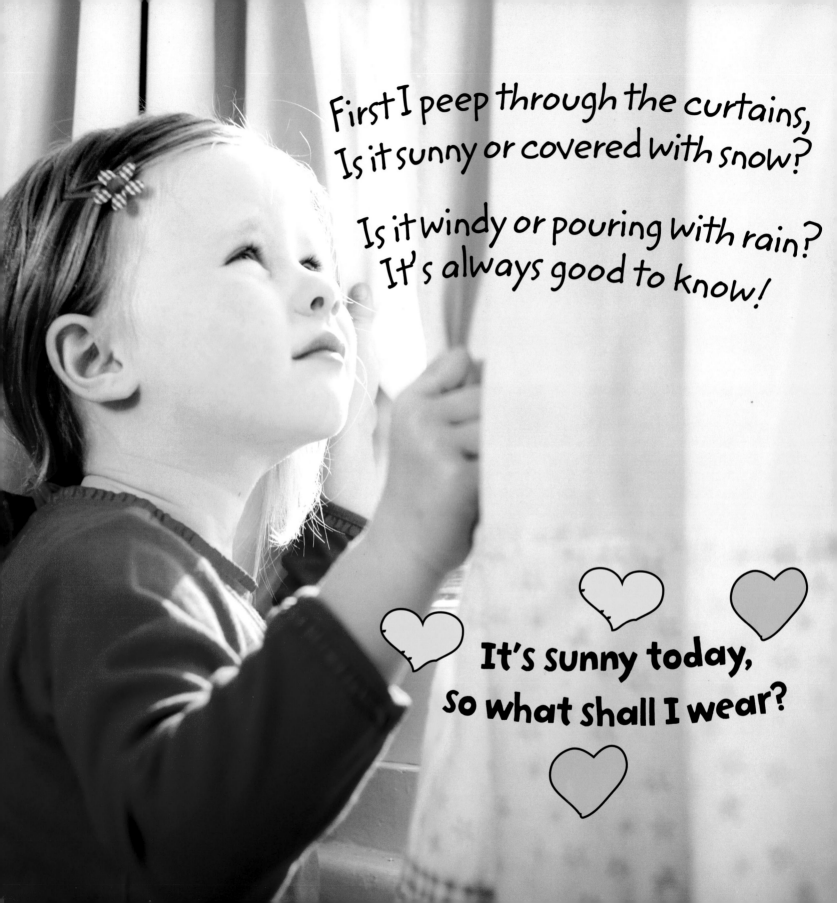

First I peep through the curtains,
Is it sunny or covered with snow?

Is it windy or pouring with rain?
It's always good to know!

It's sunny today,
so what shall I wear?

Brrr! On a snowy day I need a hat and gloves...
Phew! A sun hat is perfect for a warm day...
Splish! On a rainy day I need a raincoat and umbrella!

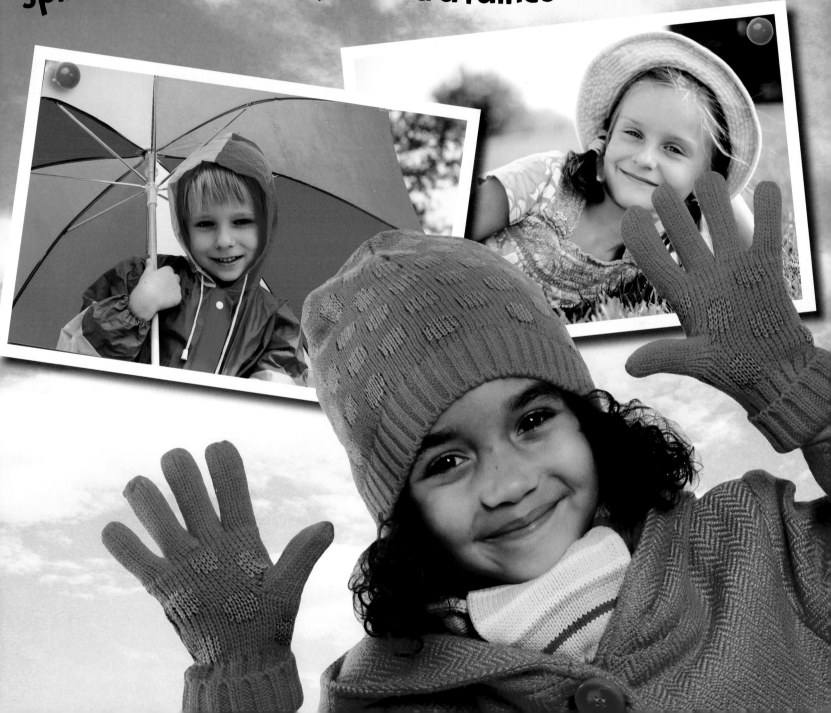

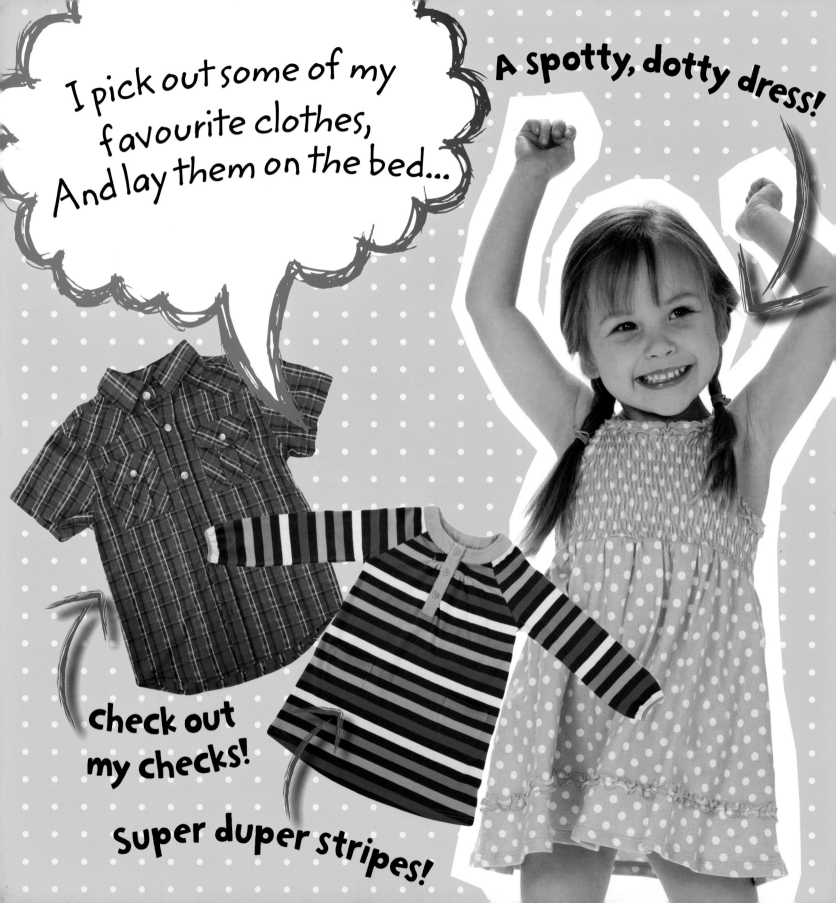

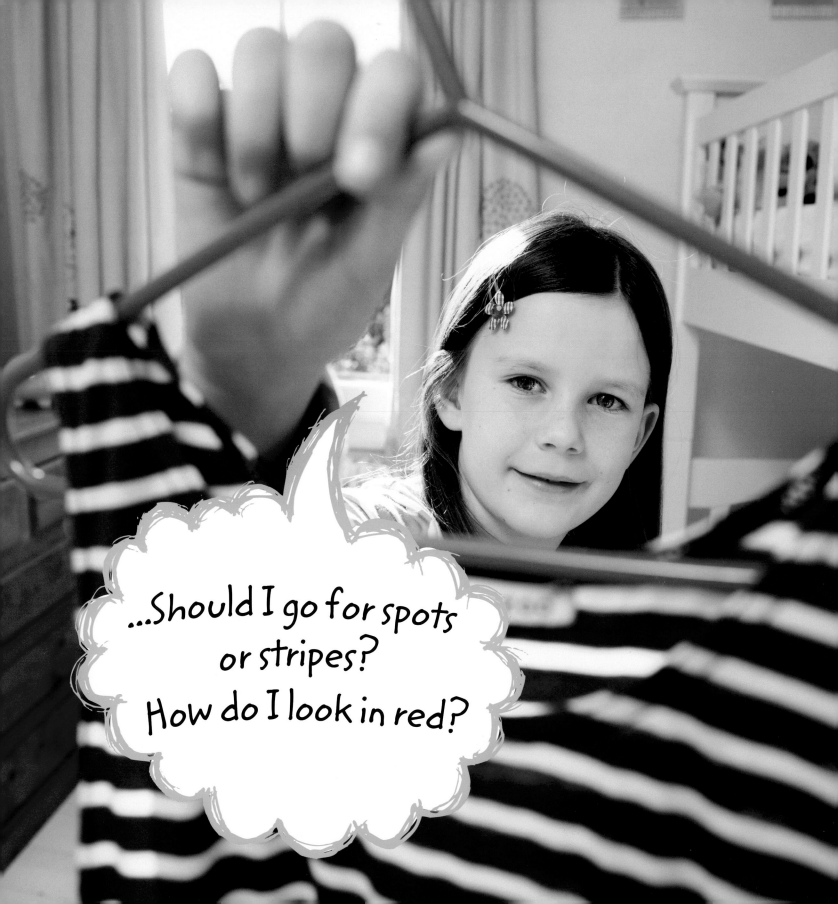

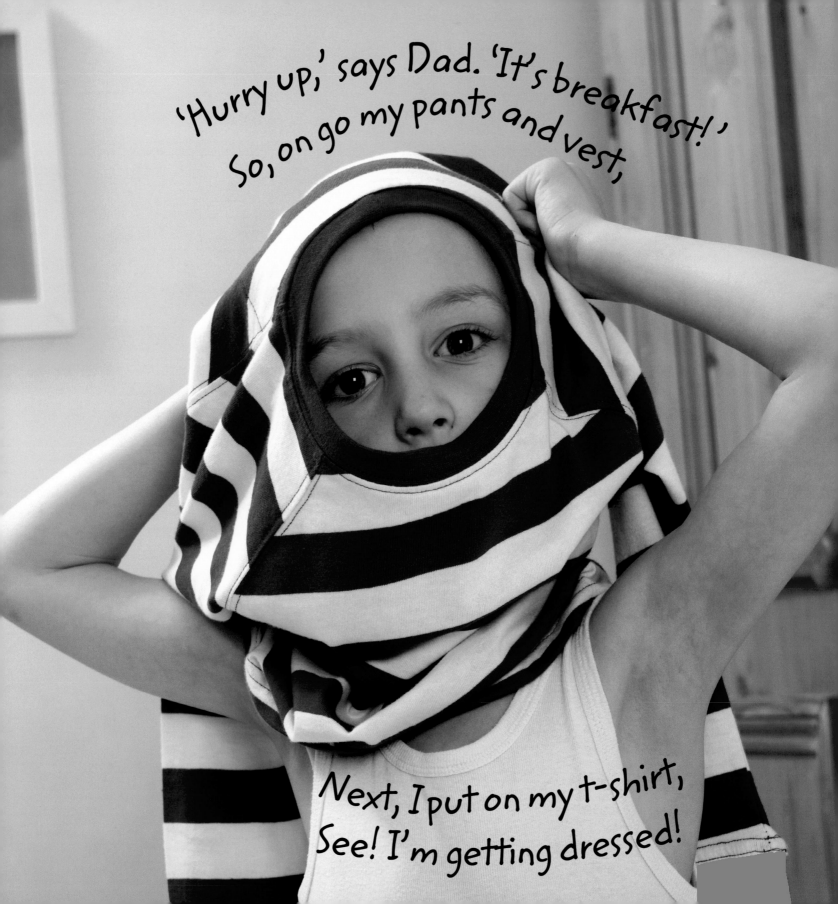

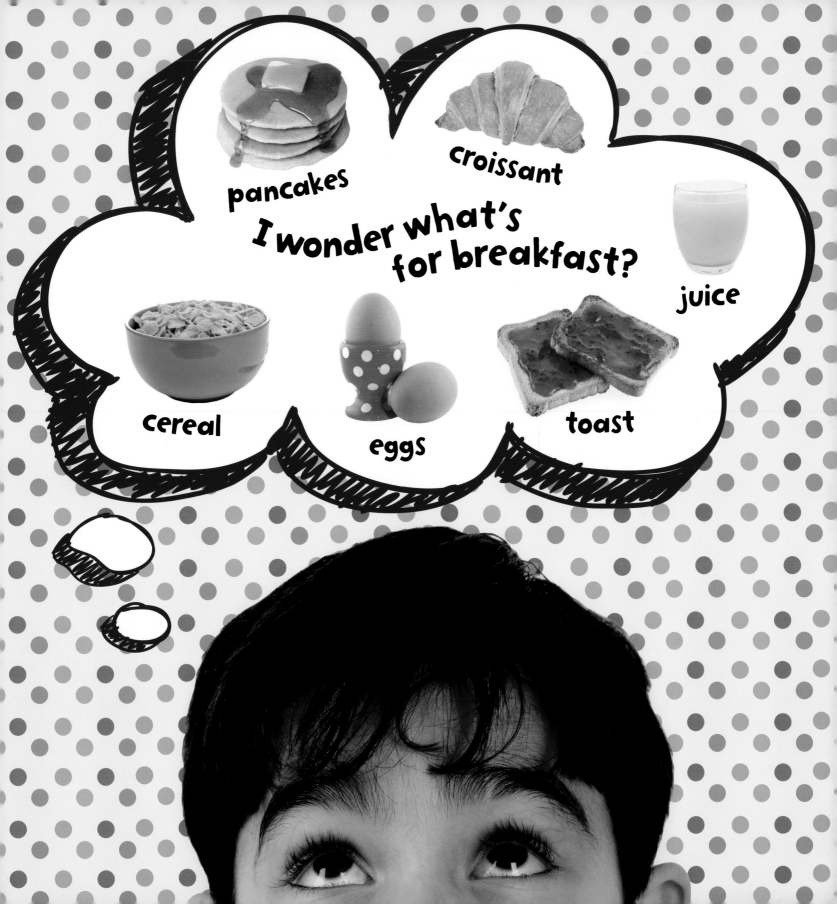

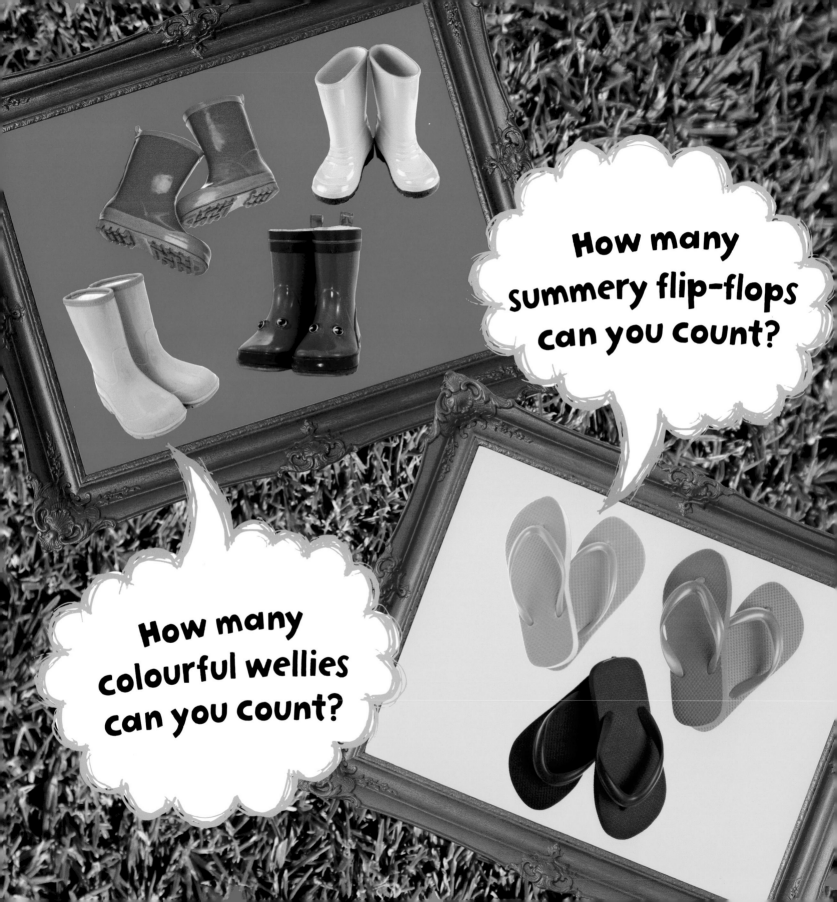

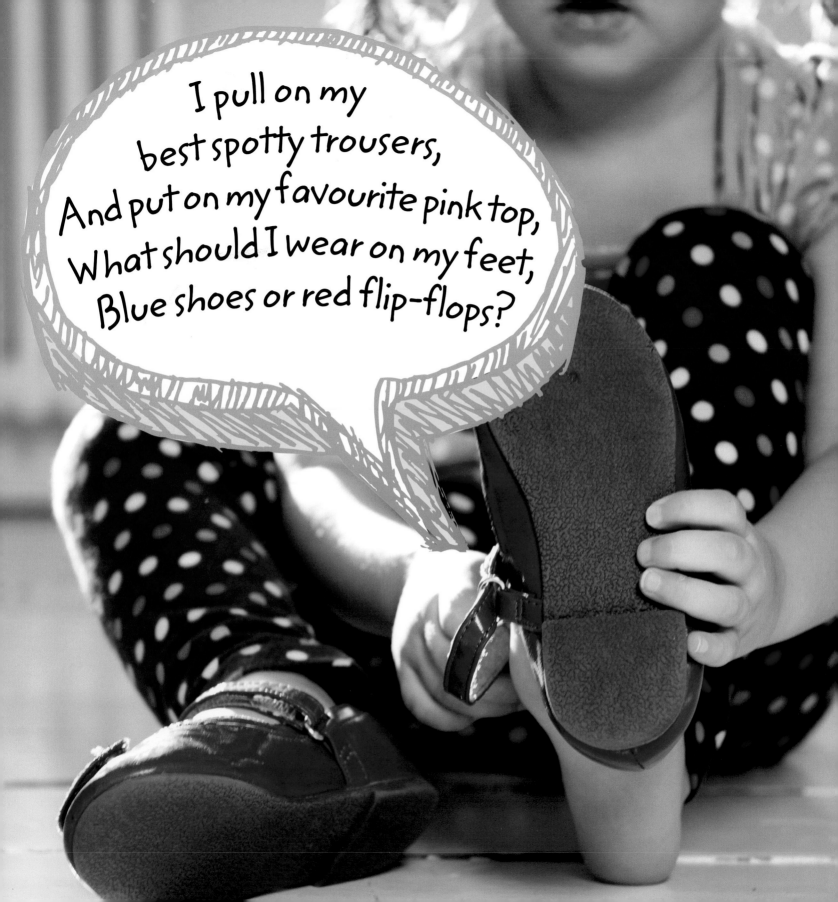

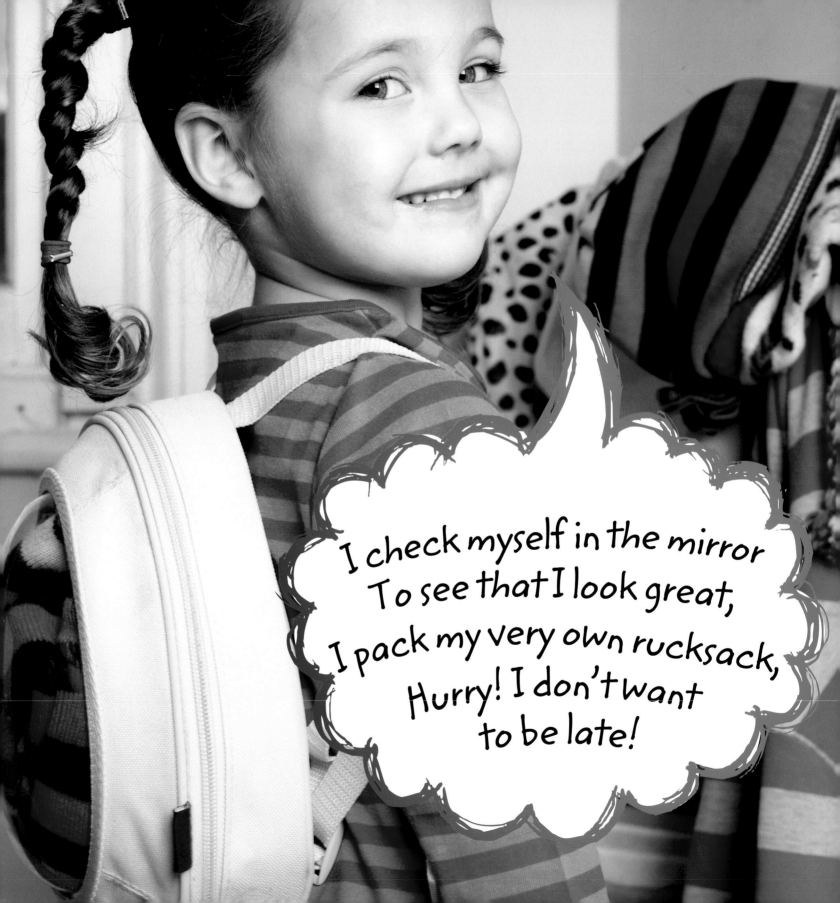

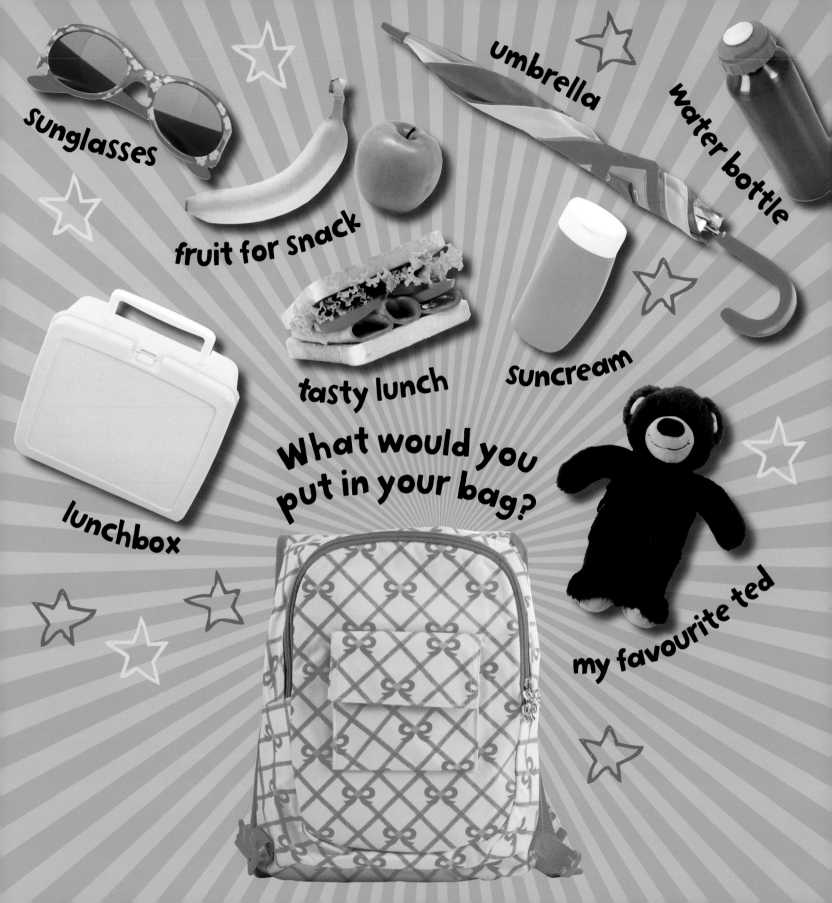

sunglasses

fruit for snack

umbrella

water bottle

tasty lunch

suncream

lunchbox

What would you put in your bag?

my favourite ted

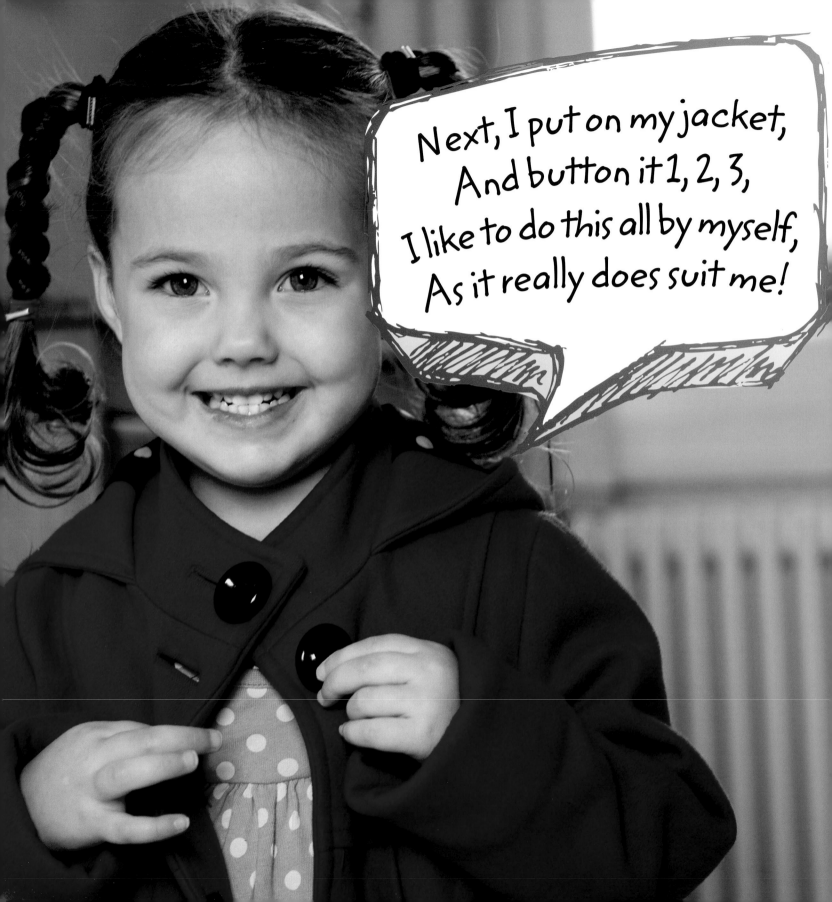

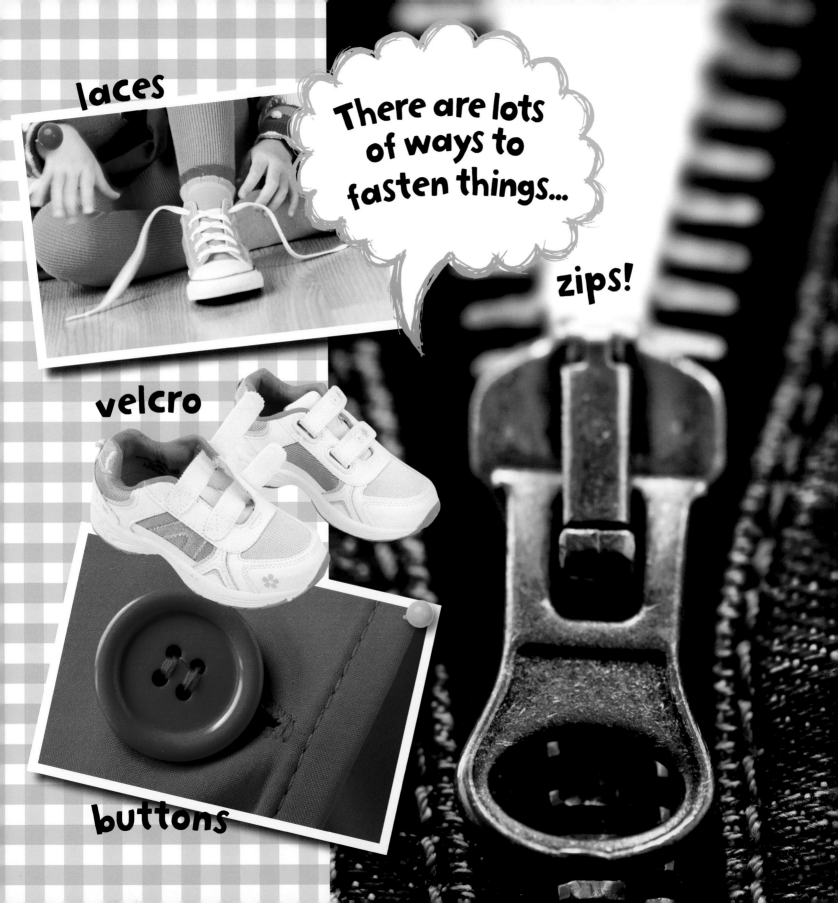

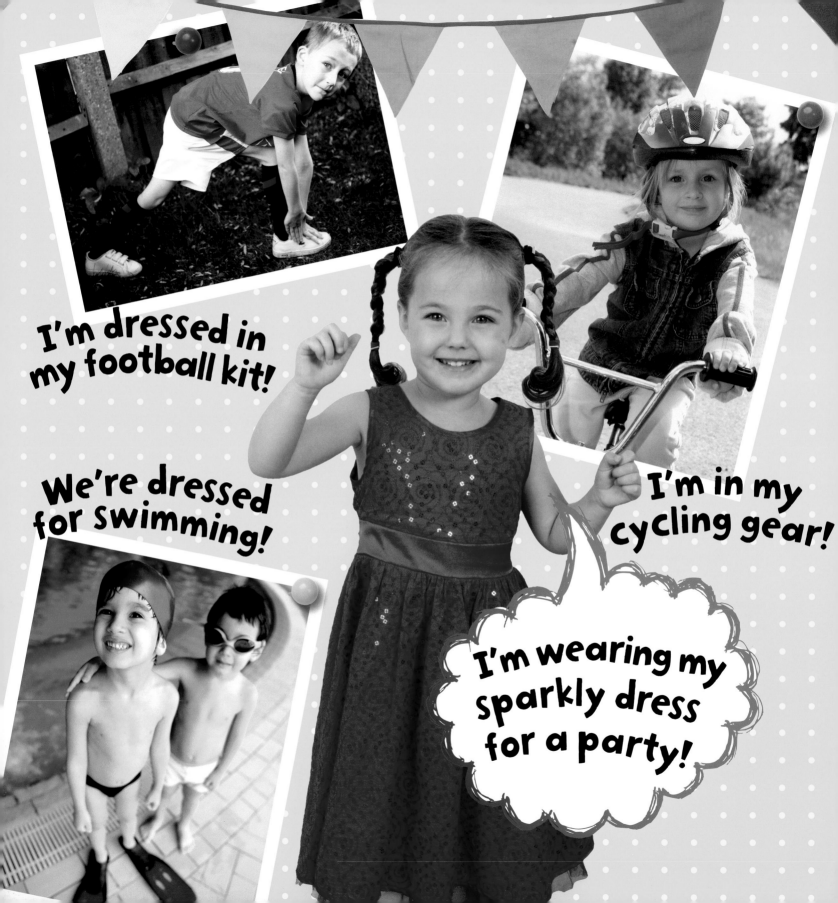

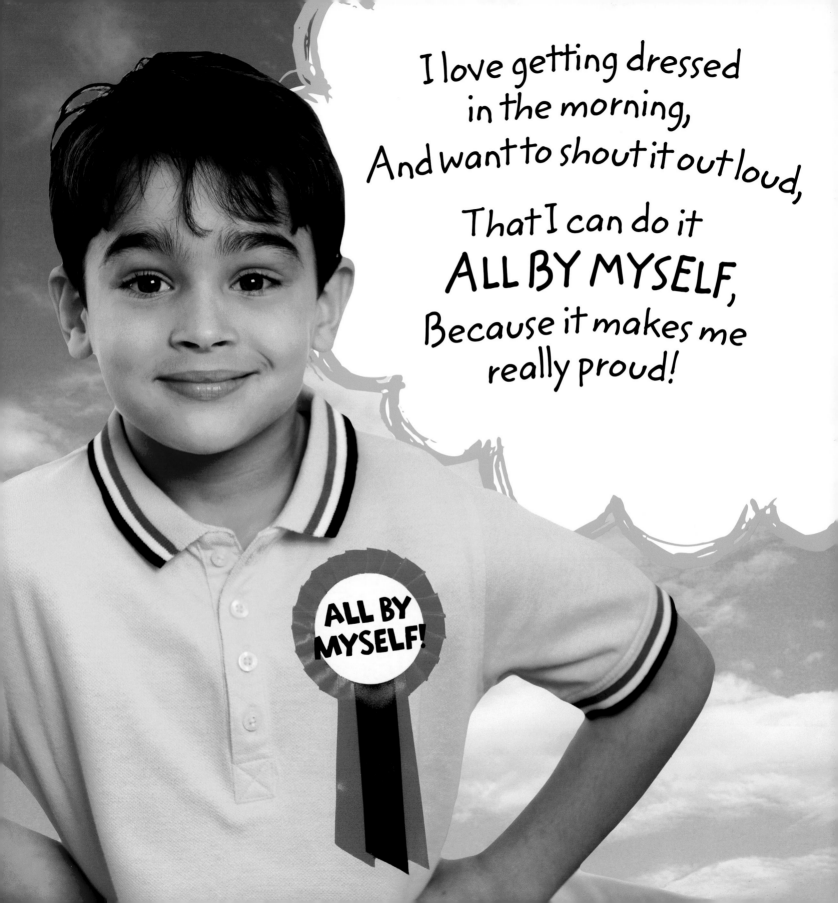

I love getting dressed
in the morning,
And want to shout it out loud,

That I can do it
ALL BY MYSELF,
Because it makes me
really proud!

Your Feelings

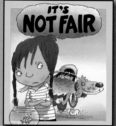
978 0 7502 2132 0

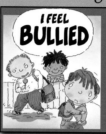
978 0 7502 2576 2

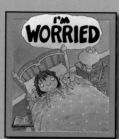
978 0 7502 2131 3

Your Emotions

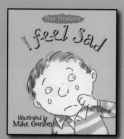
978 0 7502 1406 3

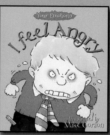
978 0 7502 1403 2

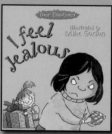
978 0 7502 1405 6

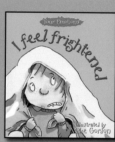
978 0 7502 1404 9

You Choose

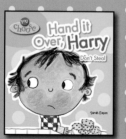
978 0 7502 6723 6

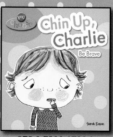
978 0 7502 6722 9

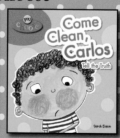
978 0 7502 6724 3

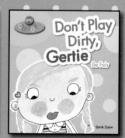
978 0 7502 6725 0